BREAKING THE SILENCE

A Comprehensive Guide to Erectile Wellness

By

Dr. Andrew Morrison

TABLE OF CONTENTS

INTRODUCTION TO ERECTILE DYSFUNCTION (ED)

Men of all ages might suffer from erectile dysfunction (ED), a complex disorder that is more common as men age. The inability to consistently get or keep an erection strong enough for satisfying sexual activity is what distinguishes it. Even though having periodic erection problems is common, ED is identified when the issue worsens over time and negatively affects a person's quality of life.

Many different physical, psychological, and lifestyle aspects might contribute to eating disorders. Cardiovascular illnesses, diabetes, hormone imbalances, neurological conditions, or anatomical problems impacting blood flow to the penis are examples of physical causes. In addition to physical illnesses already present, psychological variables such as stress, worry, depression, or relationship issues can also lead to ED and frequently exacerbate them.

Substance misuse, smoking, medication, and binge drinking can all exacerbate the problem. Lifestyle decisions, including weight, poor food, and inactivity, can also raise the chance of having ED.

A comprehensive study of the patient's medical history, a physical examination, and occasionally further procedures like blood tests, ultrasounds, or psychological evaluations to determine underlying causes are all part of the diagnosis process. The severity of the ailment and its underlying cause determine the available treatment options. These could include pharmacological treatments (such as phosphodiesterase type 5 inhibitors like Viagra), vacuum erection devices, penile implants, psychotherapy, and, in extreme situations, surgical procedures.

It's critical that people with ED consult a doctor because this condition frequently indicates an underlying health problem that has to be addressed. Enhancing general sexual health and well-being and managing the condition effectively require open conversation with partners and healthcare practitioners.

CHAPTER ONE

THE ERECTION'S ANATOMY

An erection is a complicated physiological process involving the coordinated interaction of hormone, vascular, and neurological systems. Gaining knowledge about the anatomy of erections might help one better understand the complex mechanisms involved in achieving and sustaining a hard and satisfying erection.

Nervous System Participation

Sexual excitement generates messages in the brain, particularly in areas like the hypothalamus and limbic system. These signals trigger the production of neurotransmitters, including nitric oxide.

Neurological Parasympathetic System

The smooth muscles in the erectile tissues relax as a result of nitric oxide's stimulation of the parasympathetic nervous system. This relaxation increases blood flow to the penis.

Vascular Elements

The penis has two primary arteries, the corpora cavernosa, responsible for delivering blood to the erectile tissues. Increased blood flow into these arteries is important for engorgement and the stiffness of the penis during an erection.

Two parallel chambers that stretch the entire length of the penis are called the corpora cavernosa. During an erection, the corpora cavernosa's sinusoids—small blood vessels—swell to make room for the blood influx.

Control of Hormones

Testosterone: The key hormone involved in male sex, testosterone helps to sustain libido and normal sexual function. Sufficient levels of testosterone play a role in how well the erectile process works.

Endocrine System: Hormones from the endocrine system, particularly luteinizing hormone (LH) and follicle-stimulating hormone (FSH), influence testosterone production. Normal erectile function requires hormonal balance.

Anatomy of the Penis

Corpus Spongiosum: The corpus spongiosum, which surrounds the urethra, keeps it from compressing during an erection. It also helps to make the penis more firm.

Corpora Cavernosa: The corpora cavernosa, which make up most of the penile tissue, are erectile chambers that are mostly to blame for penile stiffness. They are packed with sinusoids and blood vessels.

Erection Mechanism

Blood Engorgement: When nitric oxide is released during sexual stimulation, smooth muscle relaxes. This relaxation permits artery dilatation and increased blood flow, which causes the erectile tissues to swell.

Compression of Veins: The veins that normally carry blood away are compressed as blood fills the corpora cavernosa. The blood being trapped in the erectile tissues by this compression maintains the erection.

Comprehending the complex structure of an erection highlights the significance of a robust neural system, vascular system, and hormonal equilibrium. Any of these components can be disrupted, which highlights the need to treat erectile dysfunction with a multifaceted approach.

The physiological mechanism of erection is multifaceted, encompassing the neurological system, vascular system, and hormonal equilibrium. The release of nitric oxide is a key factor in the relaxation of smooth muscle and the enhancement of blood flow to the penis.

Function of Blood Flow: A strong and long-lasting erection depends on adequate blood flow to the erectile tissues. Any disturbance in this blood flow or the mechanisms controlling it may result in erectile dysfunction.

The Meaning and Classification of Erectile Dysfunction

The inability to obtain or sustain an erection for adequate sexual performance is known as erectile dysfunction (ED). It's critical to distinguish between primary ED, which has been present since the beginning of sexual development, and secondary ED, which develops later in life.

Clinical Definition: The chronic inability to get or sustain an erection strong enough for satisfying sexual performance is known as erectile dysfunction (ED). Based on the length and frequency of problems getting or maintaining an erection, a diagnosis is made.

Aspect Physiological: ED is characterized by abnormalities in the intricate interaction of hormonal, neurological, vascular, and psychological elements. The illness can cause anything from sporadic problems to total incapacity to achieve an erection.

Erectile Dysfunction Types

Physical or organic ED is brought on by physiological issues that impact blood flow or nerve impulses to the penis. Circulatory disorders, diabetes, and hormone abnormalities are among the conditions that can cause organic ED.

Psychogenic ED: Caused by psychological variables like stress, anxiety, or depression. Problems with emotions or mental health can interfere with a person's natural sexual response, which can result in psychogenic ED.

Mixed/Combination ED: Physical and psychological variables may play a role in many cases. Diagnosis and therapy may become more complicated when emotional elements and medical disorders are combined.

Situational ED differs from generalized ED in that the former happens in certain situations or with particular partners, while the latter is a problem that occurs in a variety of settings and with different people.

The difference between acquired and lifetime ED is that the former occurs from the moment a person reaches sexual maturity, while the latter arises later in life as a result of age or medical issues.

Complete ED is the inability to reach any level of erection, whereas partial ED is the capacity to acquire some degree of erection but not enough for satisfying intercourse.

Neurogenic ED: caused by neurological problems disrupting nerve signals to the penis. Conditions, including multiple sclerosis or spinal cord injuries, contribute to neurogenic ED.

Vasculogenic ED: associated with problems with blood flow within the penis. Accompanying conditions include venous leaks and atherosclerosis.

Comprehending the various forms of ED is essential for a precise diagnosis and customized care. Taking into account both psychological and physical aspects, a complete strategy is frequently required to address the various causes and manifestations of this disorder.

CHAPTER TWO

COMPREHENDING ERECTILE DYSFUNCTION

The inability to consistently obtain or sustain an erection strong enough for fulfilling sexual performance is known as erectile dysfunction (ED), a chronic medical issue. It entails the intricate interaction of several physiological elements, such as hormonal, vascular, neurological, and psychological ones. ED affects a man's capacity to have sex for an extended period of time and goes beyond transient issues. Underlying medical disorders like diabetes or cardiovascular disease, as well as psychological issues like stress and worry, may also be contributing causes. A thorough evaluation that takes into account lifestyle, psychological factors, and medical history is required for the diagnosis. A holistic approach to treatment frequently addresses the condition's psychological as well as physical aspects.

Reasons for Erectile Dysfunction (ED)

The complicated disorder known as erectile dysfunction (ED) is impacted by numerous psychological and physiological variables. Comprehending the underlying reasons is essential for a precise diagnosis and customized therapy. This comprehensive essay examines the various causes that lead to ED.

Factors related to the body

Cardiovascular difficulties: atherosclerosis, a build-up of plaque in arteries, can block blood flow to the penis. Hypertension and excessive cholesterol levels lead to vascular difficulties, impacting erectile performance.

Neurological Conditions: Nerve signals necessary for an erection can be interfered with by neurological conditions, including multiple sclerosis and Parkinson's disease. Damage to the spinal cord may prevent impulses from traveling from the brain to the penis.

Hormonal imbalances: Low testosterone affects libido and erectile function and is frequently linked to aging. Thyroid issues and hypogonadism are two conditions that can exacerbate hormonal imbalances that result in ED.

Factors related to lifestyle

The risk of ED is increased by tobacco smoking, which narrows blood vessels and destroys them. Smoking is a controllable risk factor, and giving it up can improve erectile function.

Abuse of alcohol and substances

Substance-induced ED may be reversible with lifestyle modifications and addiction therapy. Substance-induced ED is caused by excessive alcohol intake and substance usage, which can impair nervous system function.

Diabetes and cardiovascular disease are associated with obesity, which increases the risk of ED. Regular exercise and weight control can enhance general health and lower the incidence of ED.

Psychological Elements

Anxiety and high stress levels can cause a physiological reaction that obstructs the normal erectile function process. Situational ED may be exacerbated by relationship stress or performance anxiety.

The brain's capacity to elicit and maintain sexual excitement is impacted by depression's effects on neurotransmitter levels. In certain situations, treating underlying depression can resolve ED symptoms.

Couples therapy and open communication are crucial for treating relationship-related ED. Relationship disputes, communication issues, or a lack of intimacy can all lead to psychological ED.

Causes Associated with Medication and Treatment

ED is a possible side effect of some drugs, such as antidepressants and antihypertensive. Consulting a healthcare professional can help manage medication to reduce adverse effects.

Prostate cancer treatments such as radiation and surgery can harm blood vessels and nerves, which can affect erectile function. Post-treatment care for ED may include counselling and rehabilitation programs.

A balanced diet, frequent exercise, abstaining from tobacco and excessive alcohol use, and these lifestyle choices all promote general health and lower the risk of ED.

It's critical to monitor and manage diseases like diabetes and hypertension through routine check-ups with the doctor. The effects of these disorders on erectile function can be avoided or reduced with early intervention.

There are many different and frequently related causes of ED. Personalized treatment approaches must take into account the complexity of these elements. To effectively manage and overcome erectile dysfunction, a comprehensive strategy that addresses both psychological and physical elements is essential.

Erectile Dysfunction (ED) Risk Factors

There are numerous risk factors for erectile dysfunction (ED), including lifestyle decisions and underlying medical disorders. It is essential to identify these risk factors in order to avoid them and take early action. The main causes of ED are examined in this synopsis.

The steady decrease in testosterone levels that occurs with aging affects libido and erectile function. Although aging is not a direct cause of ED, the prevalence of ED tends to rise with age.

Reduced blood flow to the penis and vascular damage are both caused by elevated blood pressure. The negative effects of antihypertensive drugs may also affect erectile performance.

Penile blood vessels are impacted by plaque accumulation in the arteries, which reduces blood flow. Atherosclerosis is a common cause of vascular-related ED.

Disorders such as coronary artery disease can result in reduced blood flow, which can impact the penile arteries as well as the heart. The function of the erection is intimately related to cardiovascular health.

Preventing diabetes-related ED requires maintaining ideal blood sugar levels. Diabetes can harm blood vessels and nerves, impairing normal erectile function.

Factors related to lifestyle

Quitting smoking can improve general vascular health and lower the risk of ED. Tobacco use destroys blood vessels, limiting blood flow to the penis.

Overindulgence in alcohol can damage the neural system and cause ED. Moderation or complete abstinence can reduce the risk of alcohol-related ED.

Obesity is linked to a number of diseases, such as diabetes and cardiovascular problems, which exacerbate ED. Maintaining a healthy weight and lifestyle can lower the risk of ED associated with obesity.

Psychological Elements

Anxiety and high levels of stress can cause a physiological reaction that impairs regular erectile function. Reducing stress with counselling and relaxation methods can lower the risk of ED.

Depression's effects on neurotransmitter levels impact sexual arousal and satisfaction. Treating underlying sadness is crucial to preventing depression-related ED.

Adverse effects of medication

ED can occur as a side effect of some drugs, such as antihypertensive, antidepressants, and antipsychotics. Consulting a healthcare professional can help manage medications to reduce the risk of ED.

Additional Medical Conditions

Neurological disorders, including multiple sclerosis and Parkinson's disease, can affect the nerve signals necessary for an erection. Treating these disorders is critical to avoiding related EDs.

Problems with the Prostate

Prostate diseases or treatments, including radiation therapy or surgery for prostate cancer, may impact erectile dysfunction (ED). Post-treatment care may include counseling and rehabilitation therapies.

Management and Prevention

Early intervention can avoid or limit the influence of cardiovascular health, diabetes, and other risk factors on erectile function. Regular check-ups are essential for monitoring and controlling these disorders.

Knowing the ED risk factors lays the groundwork for preventative actions and focused therapies. The prevention and successful treatment of erectile dysfunction involve lifestyle changes, routine health examinations, and the treatment of underlying medical issues.

CHAPTER THREE

INDICATIONS AND MANIFESTATIONS OF IMPOTENCE (ED)

Erectile dysfunction (ED) is a disorder that can appear with varied signs and symptoms, impairing a man's ability to generate and maintain an erection for good sexual performance. The main markers that could indicate ED are examined in this book.

Having trouble getting an erection?

Not enough firmness

Having trouble getting a firm, full erection for sexual activity.

Incapacity to arouse sexuality, but not to the appropriate degree of firmness.

Variations in the Quality of Erections

There may be irregularities in the firmness and length of erections.

Recurrent episodes of poor erection quality could be a sign of deeper problems.

Difficulties in Sustaining an Erection

Early erection loss

Inability to maintain an erection during intercourse.

Early erection fading that occurs before the intercourse is finished.

Unable to Get an Erection Again

Inability to get an erection again after being interrupted or pausing for a short while during intercourse.

Ongoing difficulties keeping stiff and aroused.

Diminished Intimacy

Reduced sexual orientation

Reduced inclination or interest in having sex.

Reduction in reactivity to sexual stimuli and loss of impulsive sexual thoughts

Absence of Instinct

Lack of unplanned or spontaneous erections.

There was a noticeable drop in the frequency of morning erections.

Impact on Emotion and Psychology

Enhanced Anxiety and Stress

Higher levels of worry and concern over one's ability to perform sexually can result from having ED.

There may be problems with self-esteem and emotional suffering.

Changes in mood and depression

Persistent ED might cause sadness and a general decrease in mood.

The effect of ED on self-perception may be linked to changes in emotional well-being.

Relationship Dynamics

Problems with Intimacy

Intimate relationship tension brought on by ED might result in emotional and communication difficulties.

Relationship quality may be impacted by partner discontent or irritation.

Steer clear of sexual activity.

ED sufferers may shy away from sexual interactions out of concern that they won't be able to perform.

This avoidance can contribute to greater interpersonal difficulties.

Pain in the body

Penile Soreness or Pain

Some people with ED may feel pain or discomfort when they try to have sex.

This discomfort may be a physical sign of deeper problems that are causing ED.

Identifying the Indices of Concurrent Conditions

Early alertness to health problems

ED can detect all diabetes, hormone abnormalities, and cardiovascular problems early.

It is essential to identify and treat these underlying health problems in order to promote general wellbeing.

Getting Expert Help

Seeking expert assistance is necessary if you have persistent symptoms of eating disorders.

The root reasons can be found and addressed with the aid of early intervention and a thorough evaluation.

Understanding the emotional and interpersonal elements of ED is just as important as identifying its physical manifestations.

Effective management and treatment of erectile dysfunction require prompt recognition of the problem and obtaining expert assistance. Early intervention improves general health and well-being in addition to treating symptoms.

CHAPTER FOUR

ERECTILE DYSFUNCTION DIAGNOSIS

Men all over the world suffer from a common ailment called erectile dysfunction (ED), which is diagnosed through a combination of physical examination, lab testing, and medical history.

When diagnosing ED, it is essential to comprehend the patient's medical history. Doctors explore the following areas

Evaluating general health conditions in order to find possible systemic problems that may affect sexual function.

Identifying comorbidities such as diabetes, hypertension, and cardiovascular illnesses as known factors in ED.

Examining lifestyle decisions related to nutrition, exercise, and drug use as they may have an impact on erectile function.

Enquiring about alcohol and tobacco use since these behaviours are connected to neurological and vascular problems associated with ED.

Past sexual behaviour

Talking about how ED symptoms start and develop.

Exploring the nature of sexual relationships and the frequency of sexual activity.

History of Medication and Treatment

Examining existing prescriptions for any side effects that might be aggravating ED.

Asking about previous treatments, surgeries, or interventions relating to sexual health.

A Thorough Examination of Medical History in the Diagnosis of Erectile Dysfunction

In order to properly diagnose erectile dysfunction (ED), which is a complicated disorder with many underlying causes, a thorough medical history is essential. Comprehending the patient's medical history offers critical perspectives that enable medical practitioners to identify risk factors and design a successful treatment strategy.

Overall Health Evaluation

Examining the existence of long-term conditions like diabetes, high blood pressure, and heart disorders, which have the potential to affect the vascular and neuronal elements essential for proper erectile function,

Evaluating these conditions' length and severity in order to determine whether or not they may contribute to ED.

Inquiring about any neurological illnesses or injuries that may disrupt nerve impulses involved in the erectile process.

Assessing signs such as tingling, numbness, or changes in feeling can point to issues with the nerves.

Exploring dietary habits and the degree of physical activity, as these factors are linked to overall cardiovascular health and can influence ED.

Talking about obesity and weight control because being overweight can lead to hormone imbalances that impair sexual function.

Asking about alcohol and tobacco use, as these behaviours can both aggravate ED by affecting the vascular and neurological systems.

Talking about the usage of illegal drugs and how it could affect one's sexual health.

Compiling details about the onset and progression of the ED symptoms.

Determining the circumstances or triggers that could make the illness worse or better.

Examining the relational dynamics, stressors, and psychological elements that may be linked to eating disorders

Talking about past experiences with anxiety, depression, or other mental health issues.

History of Medication and Treatment

Examining the patient's current prescription list to find any medications that can cause ED.

Considering changes or alternatives to drugs if they are contributing to sexual dysfunction.

Finding out about any previous ED interventions or treatments, such as therapy techniques or surgeries.

Assessing the success and potential problems of earlier therapies.

Getting Expert Assistance

Recognizing how the patient views ED and how it affects their quality of life.

Promoting open dialogue to clear up any misunderstandings or worries around the illness.

Discussing the patient's expectations regarding treatment outcomes and resolving any fears or anxiety.

To diagnose ED, a thorough medical history evaluation is essential. With a comprehensive grasp of the patient's lifestyle, mental health, and physical health, it helps medical experts pinpoint the underlying issues and create individualized treatments. To guarantee a comprehensive investigation of all pertinent factors and the creation of an efficient treatment plan, open and honest communication between the patient and the healthcare professional is crucial.

Erectile Dysfunction physical Examination

An extensive physical examination aids in determining whether ED is being caused by any anatomical or physiological factors.

Inspecting the genitalia for anomalies, such as structural abnormalities or symptoms of Peyronie's disease.

Checking for fibrous plaques on the penis, which may obstruct normal blood flow during arousal, by palpating it.

Adjacent sexual features

Examining secondary sexual traits for symptoms of hormone abnormalities.

Evaluating gynecomastia presence and body hair distribution.

Assessment of Cardiovascular Conditions

Monitoring blood pressure and assessing cardiovascular health in general.

Recognizing the link between vascular problems and ED.

Examining the Body to Determine the Causes of Erectile Dysfunction and Their Underlying Factors

An important part of the diagnosis procedure for erectile dysfunction (ED) is a thorough physical examination. Healthcare providers can determine the anatomical, physiological, and circulatory factors that may be involved in the condition by conducting a thorough assessment. Here, we examine the many facets of the physical examination that was done to assess ED.

Structural Anomalies: The examination begins with a visual assessment of the genitalia to discover any structural abnormalities or irregularities.

Peyronie's Disease: The disease's symptoms, which include fibrous plaques on the penis that may cause curvature and obstruct blood flow during an erection, are of special concern.

Fibrous Plaques: The doctor can feel for fibrous plaques by palpating the penis and determining their extent and position.

Tenderness or Abnormalities: Penile tissue tenderness or abnormalities are noticed, offering information on possible ED causes.

Body Hair Distribution: Assessing the body hair distribution for any anomalies that might point to a hormonal imbalance.

Gynecomastia: Checking for the existence of this condition, which affects men and is characterized by increased breast tissue, may be related to hormonal problems that impact sexual function.

Assessment of Cardiovascular Conditions

Vascular Health: Given the close relationship between vascular problems and ED, taking a blood pressure reading is an essential first step in evaluating general cardiovascular health.

The Hypertension Connection: Determining whether or not high blood pressure is a factor in the reduced blood flow to the vaginal region.

Peripheral Artery Disease (PAD): monitoring peripheral pulses for diseases that may affect blood flow to the extremities, including the penis, such as PAD.

Assessment of Neurology

Bulbocavernosus Reflex: Evaluating the bulbocavernosus reflex, which entails pressing the head of the penis to examine the contraction of the pelvic floor muscles, Anomalies could indicate problems with the nerves.

Numbness or Tingling: examine for any genital numbness or tingling sensations, as these could be signs of nerve-related issues impairing erectile performance.

To summarize, a comprehensive assessment of the genitalia, secondary sexual characteristics, cardiovascular system, and neurological function is part of the physical examination for ED, which goes beyond a superficial assessment. This thorough method helps healthcare practitioners identify probable factors for ED and direct further diagnostic or imaging testing. For a precise and individualized diagnosis that opens the door to specialized treatment plans that target the unique underlying causes of their illness, people with ED symptoms must consult a medical practitioner.

Evaluations of Erectile Dysfunction in Lab Settings

The following laboratory tests are essential for determining the root causes and relevant factors:

Measuring testosterone levels to uncover hormonal abnormalities impacting sexual function.

Performing a lipid profile to evaluate blood pressure and any cardiovascular problems.

Blood sugar tracking

Using blood glucose testing to screen for diabetes since the disease can cause damage to the nerves and vessels.

Testing for Nocturnal Penile Tumescence (NPT)

Performing an NPT test to examine spontaneous erections during sleep, providing insights into psychogenic variables.

Tests Performed in Labs to Diagnose Erectile Dysfunction:

The diagnosis of erectile dysfunction (ED) is largely dependent on laboratory testing, which can reveal information about potential underlying medical disorders, hormonal imbalances, and cardiovascular health. In this section, we examine the many lab tests used in the overall assessment of ED.

Evaluation of Hormones

Total and Free Testosterone: To evaluate hormonal balance, measuring levels of both total and free testosterone is necessary. Insufficient testosterone levels may be a factor in ED.

Prolactin Hormone: High prolactin levels can affect erectile function and tamper with the control of testosterone.

Heart-related Markers

Cholesterol Levels: Measuring LDL, HDL, and triglyceride levels is important because excessive cholesterol can cause atherosclerosis, which narrows blood vessels in the vaginal region.

Fasting Blood Glucose Test: This test looks for diabetes, which can damage nerves and vessels and impair erectile function.

Tests of Vascular Function

Penile Doppler Ultrasound: evaluating blood flow inside the penile arteries to find any blockages or anomalies that may contribute to ED.

Testing for Nocturnal Penile Tumescence (NPT)

NPT Monitoring: Measuring erections that occur on their own as you sleep. The absence of nocturnal erections could indicate psychosocial causes of ED.

Extra Examinations

Long-Term Blood Sugar Control: Hemoglobin A1c levels should be measured, especially in diabetics, to evaluate long-term blood sugar control.

Thyroid function is evaluated by measuring TSH, T3, and T4 levels because thyroid abnormalities may impact metabolism in general and perhaps exacerbate ED.

Inflammation Marker: Assessing inflammation, which is linked to cardiovascular disease and may have an effect on erectile performance, by measuring CRP levels.

Numerous lab tests are available for erectile dysfunction (ED), with the goal of identifying any potential systemic illnesses, hormonal imbalances, or cardiovascular problems that may be linked to the disorder. These tests offer vital information that helps medical experts identify the root causes of ED and create individualized treatment regimens. Under the supervision of a healthcare professional, people with ED symptoms must have these tests completed in order to receive an accurate diagnosis and customized treatments that target the unique biochemical reasons impacting their disease. A thorough and successful management strategy for erectile dysfunction requires consulting a medical specialist.

A comprehensive evaluation, focused laboratory testing, and a detailed medical history are all part of the diagnostic process for ED. This thorough evaluation helps identify the underlying causes of ED and directs medical experts toward creating individualized treatment programs for those who are impacted by this illness. It is imperative that people with ED symptoms consult a medical practitioner for a precise diagnosis and customized treatment.

CHAPTER FIVE

OPTIONS FOR TREATMENT

There are several ways to treat erectile dysfunction (ED), from medication to lifestyle modifications. Now let's explore these categories:

A Holistic Approach to Lifestyle Modifications for Erectile Dysfunction

Making changes to one's lifestyle is essential for treating ED, as it affects both the physical and psychological components of the condition. This is a thorough examination of lifestyle modifications that can enhance erectile function:

Nutrient-Rich Foods: Place a strong emphasis on eating a diet rich in whole grains, fruits, vegetables, and lean meats.

Omega-3 Fatty Acids: Include sources like fatty fish, flaxseeds, and walnuts for their potential benefits in promoting vascular health.

Limit Processed Foods: Cut back on the intake of meals heavy in fat, sugary snacks, and processed foods, as these can aggravate cardiovascular disease and obesity.

Aerobic Exercise: Regularly engage in cardiovascular exercises that enhance cardiovascular health and stimulate blood circulation, such as walking, jogging, or cycling.

Strength Training: Include strength training activities to improve muscle health and general fitness.

Pelvic Floor Exercises: By strengthening the muscles in the pelvic floor, exercises like Kegels may help with erectile dysfunction.

Body Mass Index (BMI): Since obesity raises the risk of ED, it is important to reach and maintain a healthy BMI.

Weight Loss: For overweight people, reducing weight gradually with diet and exercise can have a good effect on sexual health.

Giving Up Smoking: Smoking can aggravate ED by damaging blood vessels. Giving up smoking enhances circulation and vascular health.

Moderating Alcohol Intake: Drinking too much alcohol might damage nerve cells and cause ED. The secret to preserving sexual health is moderation.

Mindfulness and Relaxation Techniques: To reduce stress, practice deep breathing, mindfulness, or meditation.

Quality Sleep: Make sure you get enough good sleep, since not getting enough sleep can lead to hormone imbalances and higher stress levels.

Communication: Be open and supportive in your dialogue with your partner regarding any worries you may have about ED.

Counselling or Therapy: If psychological issues like sadness or anxiety play a role in ED, get expert assistance.

Effect on Libido: Overindulging in pornography might raise irrational expectations and performance anxiety.

Balanced Sexual Perspective

A complete and all-encompassing approach to addressing erectile dysfunction is provided by lifestyle modifications. By putting these changes into practice, sexual health is addressed from a psychological and relational perspective in addition to the physical. It is advised that people with ED speak with medical professionals to create a customized plan that incorporates lifestyle changes along with other appropriate interventions for long-lasting and successful results.

Erectile Dysfunction Drugs

Medications are a popular and successful kind of treatment for erectile dysfunction (ED), offering focused approaches to improve erectile function. Now let's examine the specifics of the drugs that are frequently prescribed for ED:

Inhibitors of phosphodiesterase type 5 (PDE5)

Sildenafil (Viagra): usually taken half an hour before engaging in sexual activity.

Tadalafil (Cialis): This medication can be taken every day in lesser quantities and is well-known for its extended duration, which permits spontaneity.

Vardenafil (Levitra): similar to sildenafil, given before sexual activity.

Mode of Action

Inhibits the enzyme PDE5, increasing levels of cyclic guanosine monophosphate (cGMP).

Boosts nitric oxide's actions, encouraging the smooth muscles in the penile arteries to relax and enhance blood flow.

Management

Orally, typically only when necessary.

It is best to take this medication empty-handed for maximum absorption.

Efficiency

High success rates in achieving and sustaining erections.

Injections of the intravenosus

Alprostadil

Administration: self-administered injections directly into the side of the penis or placed as a pellet into the urethra.

Mechanism: In order to promote blood flow and cause an erection, alprostadil relaxes smooth muscles and dilates blood vessels.

Advantages

Effective for many men, even those who do not respond well to PDE5 inhibitors.

Can be used as a backup plan in cases where taking oral drugs is not appropriate.

Drawbacks

Needs self-injection, which some people may find disadvantageous.

Injection site soreness is one of the possible adverse effects.

Treatment with Testosterone Replacement

Indication

Recommended for males whose erectile dysfunction is impacted by low testosterone levels.

Forms

Available in many forms, including injections, gels, patches, or pellets implanted under the skin.

Observation

To prevent problems, regular monitoring of testosterone levels is essential.

Efficiency

Effective in cases where ED is exacerbated by low testosterone levels.

Observations and Safety Measures

Talking with the healthcare provider

Only after a comprehensive assessment by a skilled healthcare practitioner should medications for ED be recommended.

Tailored Care Programs

A patient's choice of treatment is frequently determined by their preferences, underlying ED reasons, and general health.

Interactions and Side Effects

Every medication has the potential to interact with other medications and cause negative effects. Talking about this with a healthcare professional is essential.

Certain people may not be good candidates for these medications if they have certain medical conditions or are taking certain medications.

For many people, ED medications offer practical answers that boost self-esteem and enhance quality of life in general. However, based on unique health considerations, a thorough evaluation by a medical practitioner is required to identify the best drug and dosage. The safe and efficient use of these drugs in the treatment of erectile dysfunction is ensured by open communication with a healthcare professional.

Vacuum Erection Device (VED)

A non-invasive gadget called a vacuum erection device (VED), sometimes referred to as a penis pump or vacuum pump, helps men with erectile dysfunction (ED) get and keep an erection. Let's examine the main elements, working principle, appropriate use, and factors to take into account when using vacuum erection devices:

Parts

Cylinder: a hollow tube placed over the penis.

Pump: An instrument that draws air into the cylinder by hand or with a battery.

Constriction Ring: To sustain an erection, a flexible band or ring is positioned at the base of the penis.

Action Mechanism

Production of Vacuum

The cylinder covers the flaccid penis.

A vacuum is created when the pump is turned on, drawing blood into the penis.

The Formation of Erection

An erected penis is the result of increased blood flow.

Application of Constriction Rings

The constriction ring is positioned at the base of the penis to trap blood and sustain the erection once it has been attained.

Appropriate Use

Begin with a V-shaped penis.

A flaccid penis is usually treated with this gadget.

Use lubricants. Using a lubricant with a water base at the base of the penis aids in sealing in the ideal vacuum.

Place the penis in:

Slide the penis into the cylinder, flaccid.

Produce a vacuum.

Turn on the pump to generate a suction that draws blood to the penis.

Implement a constriction ring.

After achieving an erection, position the constriction ring at the penis' base.

To avoid possible tissue damage, do not use the gadget for extended periods of time.

Benefits

Non-invasive: VEDs provide an alternative to surgery and medication for the treatment of ED.

Appropriate for a Variety of Causes: It can be used to treat ED brought on by diabetes, vascular problems, or post-prostate surgery.

Taking into account

For comfort and efficacy, the cylinder must be fitted properly.

Partner Participation:

There's a chance that partners will be involved, and communication is essential.

Safety Issues

Excessive pressure should be avoided, and usage directions should be closely followed.

Efficiency

Varying Success Rates: The underlying reasons for ED may influence success, and individual efficacy may differ.

Talking with the healthcare provider

Suggested: To make sure a VED is a safe and appropriate choice for a given set of circumstances, it is advisable to speak with a healthcare provider before utilizing one.

For males with erectile dysfunction, a mechanical, non-invasive alternative is offered via a vacuum erection device. Though it might not be appropriate for everyone, it provides a feasible choice, particularly for individuals who are unable to utilize or would rather not use drugs or intrusive treatments. As with any medical device, careful use and compliance with instructions are essential for best outcomes. For individualized counsel and direction, those thinking about a VED should speak with a healthcare professional.

Erectile Dysfunction Surgery

When various treatment options are unfeasible or inefficient for a certain individual with erectile dysfunction (ED), surgical treatments may be taken into consideration. Let's examine the several surgical approaches that can be used to treat ED:

Penile prostheses, or implants

Types

Inflatable Implants: These devices consist of inflated cylinders inserted into the penis that, when activated, cause a scrotal pump to produce regulated erections.

Malleable Implants: Manually adjustable, semi-rigid rods are inserted into the penis to provide consistent firmness.

Method

Surgically placed within the penis during a minimally invasive surgery.

Usually an outpatient procedure with a brief recuperation period.

Things to Think About

High Success Rate: Patients who receive penile implants report high levels of satisfaction.

Irreversibility: It is difficult to reverse the process, so it is important to make a thoughtful choice.

Risk of Infection: An infection could develop and necessitate immediate care.

Surgical Vascular Treatment

Indication

Appropriate for ED brought on by arterial insufficiency, in which the penis's blood supply is impeded.

Method

Surgical repair of arterial obstructions or re-routing of blood vessels to increase penile blood flow.

Usually entails arterial revascularization or bypass grafts.

Things to Think About

Success Factors: The degree and location of vascular problems affect the outcome.

Risks: There could be a chance of infection, scarring, or more blood vessel injury.

Surgery for Venous Ligation

Indication

Suitable for ED brought on by venous leaks, in which blood leaves the penis too quickly.

Method

Cutting or ligating veins surgically to stop blood flow and enable longer erections.

Things to Think About:

Particular Cases: This process is only to be used in particular situations where venous leakage is obviously a problem.

Results: Success rates differ, and in certain instances, repeating the process may be necessary.

Penile Vascularization

Indication

Considered for ED induced by pelvic trauma or vascular damage.

Method

Reconstruction or surgical repair of damaged arteries to allow the penis to receive normal blood flow again.

Things to Think About

Limited Applicability: Not every ED case is a good fit for this technique.

Effectiveness: Depending on the type and degree of artery injury, results may differ.

When alternative treatments for erectile dysfunction have failed or are not appropriate, surgical methods are usually taken into consideration. Every surgical option has a unique collection of factors, risks, and possible advantages. Choosing to have surgery should be decided after consulting with a licensed healthcare provider who can evaluate each patient's unique situation, go over possible results, and offer advice on the best course of action for treating ED.

CHAPTER SIX

THE ERECTILE DYSFUNCTION PSYCHOLOGICAL EFFECT

Beyond its outward appearance, erectile dysfunction (ED) has a profound effect on a person's psychological health. Comprehending the psychological components is essential for comprehensive care since the interplay of physical and psychological factors generates a complex landscape.

Negative Self-Perception: ED can cause feelings of inadequacy, which can have an effect on one's overall worth and self-esteem.

Decreased Confidence: The inability to get or keep an erection can lead to a decrease in confidence, which can have an impact on a number of areas of life.

Communication Issues: When a spouse finds it difficult to talk about ED, communication can break down, which strains the relationship more.

Intimacy Issues: ED may exacerbate feelings of perceived intimacy deficits, which may strain emotional bonds.

Worry of failure: This worry can exacerbate the problem by causing a vicious circle of anxiety over one's ability to perform sexually.

Pressure: The pressure to act sexually in accordance with society's expectations can heighten tension and anxiety.

Emotional Toll: Prolonged ED can cause depressive symptoms by causing emotions of melancholy, annoyance, or hopelessness.

Anxiety Disorders: Sex-related performance anxiety can develop into more widespread anxiety disorders.

Identity Threat: ED can make people revaluate their personal identities by challenging conventional ideas of what it means to be a man.

Role Expectations: When a man has ED, social expectations about his sexual performance can exacerbate feelings of failure.

Social Withdrawal: Avoiding social events because of a fear of possible humiliation or shame

Isolation: People who experience loneliness may distance themselves from close interactions.

Coping Strategies

Substance Abuse: Some people use drugs, alcohol, or other substances as a coping mechanism for the emotional pain that comes with having an eating disorder.

Avoidance Behaviours: Avoiding circumstances that may lead to sexual interactions to relieve worry and stress.

Counselling and Therapy: In order to treat the psychological components of ED, professional counselling—including sex therapy—can offer a supportive setting.

Couples treatment: Participating in treatment together helps enhance understanding and communication.

Comprehensive care requires an understanding of and attention to the psychological effects of erectile dysfunction. An individual's capacity to manage eating disorders can be greatly enhanced by acknowledging the emotional cost and obtaining the right assistance. In order to treat the complex psychological issues connected to ED, healthcare experts are essential in offering therapeutic interventions, encouraging candid communication, and giving assistance.

CHAPTER SEVEN

ERECTILE DYSFUNCTION PREVENTION AND LIFESTYLE ADVICE

Adopting a proactive strategy to prevent erectile dysfunction (ED) involves making lifestyle choices that promote cardiovascular health, maintain hormonal balance, and support overall well-being. Detailed lifestyle and preventative advice is provided below:

Place a strong emphasis on whole grains, nuts, fruits, vegetables, and lean proteins.

Include foods high in omega-3 fatty acids, such as fish and flaxseeds.

Limit your consumption of processed foods, sugary snacks, and heavy meals, as they might exacerbate obesity and cardiovascular problems.

Take part in frequent aerobic activities to strengthen your heart, such as cycling, jogging, or walking.

Incorporate strength training activities to enhance general physical well-being.

Include exercises for the pelvic floor (Kegels) to strengthen the muscles related to erection.

Keep your body mass index (BMI) within a healthy range to lower your chance of developing ED-related obesity-related problems.

Steer clear of smoke and drink in moderation.

Smoking might aggravate ED and damage blood vessels. Quitting smoking promotes vascular health.

Limit alcohol intake to moderate levels, as excessive drinking can affect nerve function and lead to ED.

To reduce stress, engage in deep breathing exercises, mindfulness, or meditation.

Make sure you get enough good-quality sleep, as insufficient sleep can lead to hormone abnormalities and elevated stress levels.

Honest Communication

Keep lines of communication open on expectations and concerns around sexual health with your spouse.

If psychological factors play a role in eating disorders, therapy or counselling may be necessary to address the underlying problems.

Frequent Medical Examinations

To treat potential cardiovascular concerns, regularly check cholesterol and blood pressure.

Regular diabetes screening to identify and treat the illness as soon as possible.

Avoid utilizing illegal drugs since they may impair one's ability to have sex.

The prevention of erectile dysfunction necessitates a comprehensive approach to general health. Lifestyle decisions that prioritize cardiovascular health, maintain a healthy weight, and manage psychological well-being contribute to sexual health. A proactive approach to avoiding ED and supporting a fulfilling and healthy sexual life must include routine check-ups, honest communication, and professional assistance as required.

CONCLUSON

$\mathbf{A}$ complex disorder having physical, psychological, and lifestyle-related components is erectile dysfunction (ED). For comprehensive treatment and efficient management, it is essential to comprehend the intricate interaction of components that contribute to ED.

Vascular Health: Issues such as atherosclerosis influence blood flow to the penis.

Neurological Factors: Nerve-related disorders that impact erection signalling

Hormonal Imbalances: Vibrations in testosterone levels or levels of other hormones that impact libido.

Effect on Self-Esteem: ED patients may experience low confidence and a poor view of themselves.

Relationship strain: problems with intimacy and communication in relationships.

Performance anxiety: the fear that one will not live up to social expectations and act sexually poorly.

Diet and Exercise: The impact of a good diet and regular exercise on promoting overall cardiovascular health.

Alcohol Use and Smoking: The detrimental effects on erectile function of alcohol drinking and smoking.

Stress Management: The importance of stress reduction approaches for psychological well-being.

Consulting medical experts to determine underlying reasons and create individualized therapy regimens

Adopting a healthy lifestyle that includes stress reduction, regular exercise, and a balanced diet.

Investigating medicative alternatives such as PDE5 inhibitors, injections, or, if required, surgical procedures

Addressing the emotional impact through counselling, therapy, and open communication with partners.

Proactively taking actions to prevent ED, including preserving cardiovascular health, controlling stress, and avoiding dangerous lifestyle choices.

Due to the complexity and subtlety of erectile dysfunction, treatment must be both comprehensive and tailored to the patient. Understanding the lifestyle, psychological, and physical components that contribute to ED enables focused therapies that enhance general wellbeing. A more fulfilling and successful sexual life can be achieved through open communication, competent advice, and an acceptance of a holistic approach to health. In order to promote a good and proactive approach to sexual health and general wellness, it is imperative that those who are experiencing ED take proactive steps to address the problem.